EASY APPROACH

TO

A HEALTHY LIFESTYLE

The Simple Secrets to a Healthy Life

BY

THOMAS C. BRUNNER

DISCLAIMER

TABLE OF CONTENTS

INTRODUCTION
The Journey to a Healthier You
Why health is wealth

Health is frequently alluded to as wealth since it is quite possibly the most important resource that we have. Without great well-being, we can't completely partake in our lives or accomplish our objectives, regardless of how rich or effective we might be in different parts of life.

Consider briefly the times when you were feeling unwell or wiped out. How could it influence your day-to-day routine? Maybe you couldn't zero in on work or partake in the organization of loved ones. Perhaps you needed to pass up occasions or exercises that you were anticipating. Or on the other hand, more regrettably, you might have needed to invest energy and cash looking for clinical regard to recuperate.

Presently ponder the times when you were healthy. You probably felt fiery, cheerful, and ready to handle anything that difficulties came in your direction. You might have had the endurance to seek after your interests, travel to new spots, or invest quality energy with friends and family. These encounters are important for what makes life satisfying and charming, and they are just conceivable when we have great well-being.

Notwithstanding the quick advantages of good well-being, there are likewise long-haul benefits. For instance, individuals who keep up with great well-being all through their lives will quite often have lower medical services expenses and better monetary soundness. They may likewise have more open doors for individual and expert development, as they are better ready to deal with pressure and adjust to new circumstances.

Then again, chronic weakness can prompt a pattern of impediments. Individuals who experience the ill effects of constant sicknesses or wounds might find it challenging to keep a task or seek after schooling or preparing. They may likewise encounter monetary difficulty because of the expense of clinical treatment and medicine.

Consequently, health is genuinely a form of wealth. It is something that we ought to esteem and focus on, similarly to our monetary assets. By dealing with our bodies and brains, we can partake in all that life brings to the table and fabricate a superior future for us as well as our friends and family.

How this book can help you achieve your health goals

"Easy approach to a healthy lifestyle" can be a priceless asset in your process in work on your wellbeing and health. This book gives pragmatic tips and systems for accomplishing your well-being objectives in a practical, simple-to-follow way.

It underlines the significance of adopting an all-encompassing strategy for well-being. This implies zeroing in on actual wellness, yet in addition tending to emotional well-being, sustenance, rest, stress the executives, and different variables that add to general prosperity. By tending to these areas, you can make a more exhaustive and powerful arrangement for accomplishing your well-being objectives.

One of the critical qualities of the "Easy approach to a healthy lifestyle" is its accentuation on effortlessness and openness. It is written in plain language and keeps away from complex clinical language, making it simple for perusers, everything being equal, to comprehend and carry out the counsel. The tips and methodologies introduced are commonsense and reasonable and can be incorporated into your everyday daily schedule without requiring a significant way of life update.

Another advantage is its attention to customization. Instead of advancing a one-size-fits-all way to deal with well-being, the writers urge perusers to recognize their exceptional necessities and inclinations and to make an arrangement that is custom fitted to their singular conditions. This improves the probability of progress, yet in addition, makes the excursion towards better well-being more agreeable and maintainable.

There's an arrangement of the scope of devices and assets to help perusers in accomplishing their objectives. These incorporate feast plans, workout schedules, and stress-decrease procedures, and that's only the tip of the iceberg. The creators likewise give direction on the most proficient method to put forth practical objectives, track progress, and remain persuaded all through the excursion.

The power of small, simple changes

Concerning making positive changes in our lives, we frequently center around enormous, emotional changes. We put forth elevated objectives, make clearing goals, and attempt to upgrade our propensities at the same time. While these methodologies can be successful now and again, they can likewise be overpowering and challenging to support over the long haul.

Little, simple changes may not seem like much all alone, however when drilled reliably over the long run, they can amount to huge enhancements in our lives. For instance, rather than focusing on a difficult drawn-out gym routine consistently, you could begin by going for a short stroll around the block every morning. Rather than attempting to wipe out all low-quality food from your eating routine without a moment's delay, you could begin by trading out one undesirable nibble for a better choice every day.

The excellence of little, simple changes is that they are a lot simpler to carry out and keep up with than large, emotional ones. They require less resolve and inspiration and can be incorporated into our day-to-day schedules without causing significant interruptions. This makes them more maintainable over the long haul and can assist us with gathering the speed we want to accomplish our objectives.

These simple changes are that they can assist us with beating the idleness and obstruction that frequently keep us from gaining ground. By beginning with little, sensible advances, we can gather certainty and speed, and start to see substantial outcomes. This can be a strong inspiration and can motivate us to continue pushing ahead, in any event, whenever troubles arise.

Little, and basic changes ought to be considered carefully. By zeroing in on making steady upgrades in our propensities and schedules, we can make forward movement and fabricate the strength we want to accomplish our objectives. So go ahead and begin little - each certain step you take, regardless of how little, can carry you nearer to the better, more joyful life you merit.

With regards to rolling out sure improvements in our lives, we frequently center around enormous, sensational changes. We put forth grand objectives, make clearing goals, and attempt to redesign our propensities at the same time. While these methodologies can be viable now and again, they can likewise be overpowering and challenging to support over the long haul.

Little, basic changes may not seem like much all alone, however, when drilled reliably over the long haul, they can amount to critical enhancements in our lives. For instance, rather than focusing on an overwhelming extended exercise routine consistently, you could begin by going for a short stroll around the block every morning. Rather than attempting to take out all low-quality food from your eating regimen without a moment's delay, you could begin by trading out one undesirable nibble for a better choice every day.

CHAPTER 1
THE FOUNDATION OF A HEALTHY LIFESTYLE: MINDSET
What is a healthy lifestyle?

A healthy lifestyle is a way of living that incorporates habits and behaviors that promote physical, mental, and emotional well-being. It involves making conscious choices that support overall health and well-being, such as eating a balanced and nutritious diet, engaging in regular physical activity, getting enough sleep, managing stress effectively, and avoiding harmful habits such as smoking and excessive alcohol consumption.

A healthy lifestyle also involves taking care of mental and emotional health, such as engaging in activities that promote relaxation and enjoyment, building strong social connections, and seeking support when needed. It may also involve adopting healthy habits such as practicing mindfulness and meditation, engaging in creative pursuits, and pursuing personal growth and development.

The importance of mindset in achieving a healthier lifestyle

Developing a healthy lifestyle is a journey that demands commitment and perseverance. However, one of the most crucial variables that can dramatically affect your success in achieving a better lifestyle is your thinking. The way you think about health and well-being can either empower or hinder your progress toward your goals.

Here are some ways in which having a positive and growth-oriented mentality can support your efforts toward a healthy lifestyle:

1. Motivation: A positive mindset can help you stay motivated and devoted to your goals. When you trust in your abilities to make great changes, you are

more likely to take action and follow through on your objectives.

2. Resilience: A healthy lifestyle is not simply about eating properly and exercising regularly. It also requires controlling stress, getting proper sleep, and prioritizing self-care. With a positive perspective, you may create resilience and bounce back from setbacks or problems that may emerge along the path.

3. Self-efficacy: A healthy attitude can also boost your self-efficacy, which is your belief in your capacity to achieve your goals. When you have confidence in yourself and your ability to make positive changes, you are more inclined to continue in the face of hurdles and disappointments.

4. Focus: A positive mindset can also help you stay focused on your goals and prioritize your health and wellness. When you have a clear vision of what you want to achieve, you can better match your everyday routines and actions with your long-term goals.

5. Mind-body connection: Finally, having a good mentality helps increase the mind-body connection, which is the relationship between your thoughts, emotions, and physical health. When you approach health and wellness with a positive and growth-oriented mindset, you can better tune in to your body's requirements and make decisions that promote your overall well-being.

Benefits of a healthy lifestyle

Adopting a healthy lifestyle can give several benefits for physical, mental, and emotional well-being. Here are some of the benefits of a healthy lifestyle:

1. Reduced risk of chronic diseases: A healthy lifestyle can help reduce the risk of chronic diseases such as heart disease, stroke, diabetes, and some malignancies. By keeping a healthy weight, eating a nutritious diet, engaging in regular physical activity,

and avoiding hazardous habits such as smoking, you can minimize your risk of acquiring these diseases.

2. Improved mental and emotional health: A healthy lifestyle can also support good mental and emotional health, including reducing stress, anxiety, and depression. Engaging in activities that encourage relaxation, social connection, and personal growth can assist increase overall well-being.

3. Increased energy and productivity: By keeping a healthy lifestyle, you can improve energy levels and enhance productivity. Regular physical exercise, appropriate sleep, and a balanced diet can give the necessary fuel for the body and mind to work optimally.

4. Improved sleep quality: A healthy lifestyle can also increase sleep quality, leading to greater physical and mental health. Regular physical exercise, relaxation techniques, and a good diet can all contribute to better sleep.

5. Enhanced quality of life: A healthy lifestyle can assist boost overall quality of life, by supporting good physical, mental, and emotional health. By adopting healthy habits and behaviors, you can have a stronger feeling of well-being, enhanced relationships, and increased enjoyment.

CHAPTER 2
NOURISHING YOUR BODY: NUTRITION AND HYDRATION
The basics of healthy nutrition and hydration

Maintaining a healthy lifestyle demands a foundation of balanced eating and hydration. By nourishing your body with nutrient-dense foods and staying hydrated, you can create the foundation for a healthier lifestyle. In this post, we will discuss simple and easy-to-follow strategies for healthy nutrition and hydration, including the benefits of a balanced diet, the importance of portion control, and the function of water in general health. With these guidelines, you may make sensible choices thereby taking the first steps towards a healthier, happier you

1. Plan Ahead:

The first step to making sensible eating choices is to plan. Meal planning can help you choose nutritious and balanced meals that are packed with necessary nutrients. Take some time to plan your meals for the week, including snacks, and develop a grocery list. This can help you avoid impulse purchases and ensure that you have healthy options easily available.

2. Read Labels:

Reading labels is vital in making healthy food decisions. Be sure to study the ingredients and nutritional information before purchasing any packaged items. Look for foods that are low in sugar, saturated fats, and sodium, and high in fiber and protein.

3. Choose Whole Foods:

Whole foods are foods that are little processed and include no added sugars, salt, or fats. Examples of entire foods include fruits, vegetables, whole grains, and lean proteins. These foods are nutrient-dense, meaning they include vital vitamins, minerals, and fiber.

4. Focus on Color:

Eating a variety of colored fruits and vegetables can ensure that you are getting a wide range of nutrients. Different hues in fruits and vegetables correspond to different vitamins, minerals, and antioxidants. So, try to include a variety of hues in your diet, such as green leafy vegetables, orange carrots, red berries, and blueberries.

5. Eat a balanced diet:

A balanced diet includes a range of foods from all dietary groups, such as fruits, vegetables, whole grains, lean proteins, and healthy fats. This ensures that your body obtains all the vital nutrients it needs to function effectively.

6. Portion control:

Controlling your portion sizes is vital for keeping a healthy weight. Use smaller dishes, measure your food, and avoid eating until you are stuffed.

7. Avoid processed meals:

Processed foods are generally heavy in calories, sugar, salt, and harmful fats, which can lead to weight gain and health problems. Instead, pick full, unprocessed foods as much as possible.

8. Stay hydrated:

Drinking enough water is vital for general health. It helps regulate body temperature, transmit nutrients, and cleanse out impurities. Aim to drink at least 8-10 cups of water every day.

9. Limit sugary drinks:

Sugary drinks such as soda and energy drinks can contribute to weight gain and health problems such as diabetes and heart disease. Instead, pick water, herbal tea, or low-calorie drinks.

10. Watch your salt intake:

Too much salt can contribute to high blood pressure and other health problems. Limit your salt intake by avoiding processed foods, and use herbs and spices to add flavor to your meals.

11. Practice moderation:

It's alright to enjoy snacks and indulgences periodically. Practice moderation and enjoy them in modest portions.

By adopting these basic concepts of proper eating and hydration into your lifestyle, you may maintain optimal health and wellness. Remember to make tiny, progressive changes to your nutrition and hydration habits, and focus on progress, not perfection. A healthy lifestyle is a journey, not a destination, so be patient and persistent in your efforts.

The role of macronutrients and micronutrients in the body

Macronutrients and micronutrients are like the superheroes of the human body, each with their particular set of powers and talents. Just like a superhero team needs a varied range of powers to keep the world safe, the body requires both macronutrients and micronutrients to function efficiently.

Macronutrients are the energy providers of the body, and they are vital for powering daily activities. Carbohydrates are like rapid sprinters, giving the quick bursts of energy needed for short-term activity. Proteins are the muscle builders, needed for repairing and developing tissues, just as how a construction worker is essential for building strong, durable buildings. Fats are like endurance runners, providing long-term energy stores for the body to dip into when needed.

Micronutrients, on the other hand, are like the support squad, supplying crucial functions needed for the superheroes to fulfill their missions. Vitamins are the boosters, giving the needed chemicals that help with functions such as maintaining a healthy immune system, like a shield against hazardous intruders. Minerals are the stabilizers, helping to control biological functions such as fluid balance, like the foundation of a house that maintains it solid and robust.

Together, macronutrients and micronutrients make a powerful team that works together to keep the body healthy and working effectively. A balanced diet rich in both macronutrients and micronutrients is vital for maintaining good health.

The benefits of hydration and how to stay hydrated

Hydration is vital for overall health and well-being. It helps to regulate body temperature, carry nutrients and oxygen to cells, and drain away pollutants from the body. Dehydration, on the other hand, can lead to weariness, headaches, dizziness, and other health concerns.

The best approach to staying hydrated is by drinking adequate fluids, especially water, throughout the day. How much water you require might vary depending on factors such as age, gender, activity level, and climate. As a general guideline, adults should strive to drink at least 8-10 glasses of water every day, or more if they are active or live in hot, dry locations.

In addition to water, you can also hydrate with various fluids such as herbal tea, 100% fruit juice, coconut water, and milk. However, be wary of drinks with additional sugar, caffeine, or alcohol, as they can dehydrate the body.

Eating foods with high water content, such as fruits and vegetables, can also help keep you hydrated. Foods like watermelon, cucumber, celery, and lettuce are highly hydrating.

Staying hydrated is vital for sustaining overall health and well-being. Drinking adequate water and other fluids throughout the day, eating hydrating meals, and being careful of drinks that can dehydrate the body will help you keep hydrated and get the benefits of hydration.

CHAPTER 3
THE POWER OF MOVEMENT: EXERCISE AND PHYSICAL ACTIVITY

Understanding the value of physical activity for overall health

Physical activity is a vital component of a healthy lifestyle. Engaging in regular physical activity can help prevent and manage a wide range of chronic conditions, including cardiovascular disease, type 2 diabetes, and certain types of cancer. In addition to these physical health benefits, physical activity can also boost mental health and overall well-being.

One of the most significant benefits of physical activity is its impact on cardiovascular health. Regular exercise can assist improve cardiovascular health by strengthening the heart and reducing the risk of developing heart disease. Physical activity can also help lower blood pressure, reduce cholesterol levels, and improve blood sugar control, all of which are vital for maintaining excellent heart health.

In addition to its impact on cardiovascular health, physical activity can also help prevent and control type 2 diabetes. Exercise can help enhance insulin sensitivity, allowing the body to better regulate blood sugar levels. Regular physical activity can also help avoid obesity, which is a key risk factor for developing type 2 diabetes.

Physical activity can also play a significant role in preventing certain types of cancer. Studies have indicated that engaging in regular physical activity can help reduce the risk of acquiring breast, colon, and lung cancer. Exercise can help reduce inflammation in the body, which may have a role in the development of some types of cancer.

In addition to its physical health benefits, physical activity can also have a good impact on mental health. Exercise has been demonstrated to alleviate symptoms of sadness and anxiety, improve mood, and enhance cognitive performance. Regular physical activity can also assist enhance sleep quality, which is vital for general health and well-being.

Despite these benefits, many people do not engage in regular physical activity. This may be due to a lack of time, finances, or motivation. However, even tiny levels of physical activity can have a good impact on health. The World Health Organization recommends that individuals engage in at least 150 minutes of moderate-intensity aerobic physical activity or 75 minutes of vigorous-intensity aerobic physical activity every week.

All these demonstrate that physical activity is an essential component of a healthy lifestyle. Regular exercise can help prevent and manage chronic diseases, improve cardiovascular health, reduce the risk of getting some forms of cancer, and enhance mental health and overall well-being. It is crucial to make physical activity a priority in daily life to reap the many benefits it has to offer.

Different types of exercise and how to include them into your routine

There are three basic types of exercise: aerobic, strength, and flexibility. Each type offers various health benefits and may be incorporated into your hectic lifestyle in different ways.

☐ Aerobic activity: This sort of exercise boosts your heart rate and breathing, promoting cardiovascular health and burning calories. Examples include brisk walking, jogging, cycling, swimming, and dancing. To add aerobic exercise into your routine, try to arrange at least 30 minutes of moderate-intensity activity, such as brisk walking, most days of the week. You can divide up this time into smaller intervals throughout the day, such as 10 minutes in the morning, afternoon, and evening.

☐ Strength training: This sort of exercise involves working your muscles with resistance, such as lifting weights or utilizing resistance bands. Strength exercise can help build muscle, boost bone density, and improve metabolism. To add strength training into your program, aim to complete exercises that target all major muscle groups, such as push-ups, squats, lunges, and bicep curls, two to three times per week. You may do these workouts at home or a gym.

☐ Flexibility training: This sort of exercise improves the range of motion in your joints and can help prevent injuries. Examples include stretching, yoga, and Pilates. To add flexibility training into your program, strive to stretch all main muscle groups after each workout or activity session. You can also attend a yoga or Pilates session once or twice a week.

To make exercise a regular part of your routine, start by setting reasonable goals and progressively increasing the duration and intensity of your workouts. Find activities that you enjoy and that match your lifestyle, such as walking with a friend, joining a sports team, or taking a dance class. You can also try incorporating physical activity into your everyday routine, such as taking the stairs instead of the elevator, parking farther away from your destination, or taking a stroll during your lunch break. Remember to contact your doctor before starting any new exercise program.

Creating a personalized exercise plan that suits your lifestyle

Creating a tailored exercise plan requires creating a fitness program that matches your lifestyle and fulfills your demands and goals. Here are some steps you may take to establish an exercise regimen that works for you:

1. Determine your fitness goals: Figure out what you want to achieve with your fitness regimen. Are you wanting to lose weight, build muscle, enhance your cardiovascular health, or simply stay active?

2. Assess your present fitness level: Take stock of your present fitness level, including your strengths and limitations. Consider things including your age, weight, current fitness level, and any health risks.

3. Choose activities that you enjoy: Select exercises that you enjoy performing and that fit with your lifestyle. This could include activities like

swimming, cycling, yoga, strength training, or team sports.

4. Set a realistic timetable: Determine how much time you can commit to exercise each week and build a schedule that matches your lifestyle. Be realistic about the amount of time you can spend to exercise and develop your plan around that.

5. Create a balanced routine: Aim to include a variety of exercises that engage different muscle groups and give a combination of cardiovascular and strength-training activities.

6. Monitor your improvement: Keep track of your progress by routinely evaluating your fitness level and assessing how you feel. Adjust your plan as needed to ensure that you are continuing to make progress toward your goals.

Remember, the key to establishing a great workout regimen is to make it pleasurable, sustainable, and achievable.

CHAPTER 4
MANAGING STRESS: MINDFULNESS AND SELF-CARE

Understanding the impact of stress on physical and mental health

Stress is a natural response to tough conditions, but when it becomes chronic or protracted, it may have a dramatic influence on both our physical and mental health. The effects of stress can be both immediate and long-term, impacting practically every system in the body.

Physically, stress can impair the immune system, leaving us more prone to illness and disease. It can also increase the risk of cardiovascular disorders such as high blood pressure and heart disease. Stress can induce tension headaches, intestinal problems, and sleep abnormalities, which can further exacerbate physical health issues.

Mentally, stress can alter our mood, thoughts, and conduct. It can create emotions of anxiety, irritation, and despair, and can lead to negative self-talk and feelings of hopelessness. Stress can also interfere with our capacity to concentrate and make judgments, making it harder to perform effectively at work or school.

Chronic stress can also increase the chance of acquiring mental health disorders such as anxiety and depression. It can potentially contribute to the development of more serious illnesses like post-traumatic stress disorder (PTSD).

The influence of stress on physical and mental health is interconnected, with each affecting the other. For example, stress-related physical symptoms can lead to greater anxiety, while chronic stress can produce physical health problems that contribute to feelings of depression or hopelessness.

To lessen the impact of stress on both physical and mental health, it is vital to adopt stress management practices such as exercise, meditation, and seeking social support. Additionally, obtaining professional treatment from a therapist or healthcare provider can be effective in managing stress-related physical and mental health difficulties.

By recognizing the impact of stress on both physical and mental health and taking proactive steps to manage it, we can improve our overall well-being and lead happier, healthier lives.

Mindfulness techniques for stress reduction and relaxation

Mindfulness is a form of meditation that involves paying attention to the present moment without judgment. Practicing mindfulness can help reduce stress and increase relaxation. Here are some techniques:

1. Body Scan Meditation: Lie down or sit comfortably, close your eyes, and take a few deep breaths. Then, starting at your toes, focus your

attention on each part of your body, moving up to your feet, ankles, calves, knees, thighs, hips, abdomen, chest, arms, shoulders, neck, and head. Notice any sensations, tension, or discomfort in each region, and breathe deeply into that portion of your body, allowing it to relax and release tension.

2. Mindful Breathing: Sit comfortably with your back straight, and focus your attention on your breath. Notice the sensation of the breath as it enters and departs your body. You can count your breaths if it helps you stay focused. If your mind wanders, simply return your attention to your breath without judgment.

3. Walking Meditation: Find a quiet spot to stroll slowly and attentively. Focus on each step, experiencing the sensation of your feet touching the earth. Pay attention to your surroundings, employing all of your senses to take in the sights, sounds, smells, and textures of your environment.

4. Visualization: Close your eyes and visualize yourself in a serene, calming area, such as a beach, forest, or summit. Use your imagination to build a detailed image of your environment, including the colors, sounds, and sensations. Focus on your breath as you visualize yourself in this serene place.

5. Gratitude Practice: Take a few moments each day to focus on the things you're grateful for. Write them down in a journal, or simply think about them. Focusing on the positive can help shift your mindset and reduce stress.

These are just a few examples of mindfulness techniques for stress reduction and relaxation. Remember, the goal is to be present at the moment, without judgment, and to allow yourself to completely experience each sensation and emotion as it emerges.

Self-care strategies for promoting a healthier mindset

Self-care is a crucial element in promoting a healthier mentality. It involves taking care of your physical, emotional, and mental health needs to sustain overall well-being. Self-care practices differ from person to person, but here are some creative and practical approaches to foster a better mentality.

1. Exercise regularly: Exercise is a fantastic approach to improving your physical and mental health. It helps to relieve stress, improve mood, and boost self-confidence. Regular exercise also helps to maintain a healthy weight, minimize the risk of chronic diseases, and promote better sleep.

2. Practice mindfulness: Mindfulness is being present at the moment and paying attention to your thoughts and feelings without judgment. It helps to relieve stress, anxiety, and depression,

and promotes overall well-being. You can develop mindfulness through meditation, breathing exercises, or simply by taking a few seconds to focus on your breath.

3. Get enough sleep: Sleep is vital for sustaining excellent physical and mental health. It helps to relieve stress, improve mood, and boost cognitive function. Aim for 7-9 hours of sleep each night, and maintain a consistent sleep regimen to assist promote healthy sleep habits.

4. Eat a nutritious diet: A healthy diet is vital for sustaining good physical and mental health. Eat a mix of fruits, vegetables, whole grains, lean proteins, and healthy fats to ensure that you are getting all the nutrients your body needs. Avoid processed foods, sugary drinks, and excessive alcohol consumption.

5. Take breaks and emphasize self-care: It's crucial to take breaks and prioritize self-care, even if you have a busy schedule. Make time for

hobbies, social activities, and relaxation. Schedule self-care activities like yoga, massage, or a spa day into your routine.

6. Connect with others: Connection with others is vital for maintaining healthy mental health. Spend time with friends and family, join a social organization or community, or consider talking to a therapist or counselor if you need more assistance.

7. Set realistic goals: Setting realistic goals is a wonderful strategy to build a healthier mentality. Make a list of achievable goals, and divide them down into doable chunks. Celebrate your victories along the journey, and be nice to yourself if you meet setbacks.

8. Practice gratitude: Practicing gratitude means focusing on the positive parts of your life and being thankful for what you have. It helps to boost mood, reduce stress, and promote a sense of well-being. Consider keeping a thankfulness

diary, and write down three things you are glad for each day.

Self-care is vital for promoting a healthier mentality. Incorporating these innovative and practical self-care practices into your daily routine can help to reduce stress, improve mood, and boost overall well-being. Remember to be nice to yourself, prioritize self-care, and seek support if required.

CHAPTER 5
THE IMPORTANCE OF REST AND RECOVERY: SLEEP AND RELAXATION
The benefits of quality sleep and relaxation

Sleep and relaxation are vital for maintaining healthy physical and mental health. Here are some innovative ways to explain the benefits of quality sleep and relaxation:

1. Improved physical health:

Quality sleep and relaxation contribute to promoting greater physical health. During sleep, the body repairs and regenerates tissues improves the immune system, and regulates hormones. Relaxation helps to relieve muscle tension, regulate blood pressure, and improve digestion.

2. Better mental health:

Quality sleep and relaxation also boost mental health. Sleep helps to improve cognitive function, memory, and focus. Relaxation helps to relieve stress, anxiety, and sadness.

3. Increased creativity and productivity:
Getting adequate quality sleep and relaxation can enhance creativity and productivity. When well-rested and relaxed, you are more likely to be focused, attentive, and able to think creatively. This can lead to higher productivity at work or in other aspects of your life.

4. Improved connections:
Quality sleep and relaxation can also improve your relationships. When you are well-rested and calm, you are more patient, empathic, and able to communicate effectively. This can help to enhance ties with family, friends, and coworkers.

5. Reduced risk of chronic diseases:

Chronic sleep deprivation and stress can increase the chance of acquiring chronic diseases such as diabetes, heart disease, and obesity. Quality sleep and relaxation can assist to lower this risk by increasing general health and reducing stress levels.

6. Improved athletic performance:
Quality sleep and relaxation can also boost athletic performance. Sleep helps to increase muscular repair, reaction time, and coordination. Relaxation can help to reduce muscle tension, enhance flexibility, and lessen the chance of injury.

Common sleep disorders and how to address them
Several common sleep problems can have a substantial impact on a person's general health and well-being. These include:

1. Insomnia: Insomnia is characterized by trouble falling asleep or staying asleep. It can lead to daytime weariness, mood problems, and difficulties concentrating.

2. Sleep Apnea: Sleep apnea is a condition in which a person stops breathing for short durations during sleep. This can induce loud snoring, daytime weariness, and an increased risk of high blood pressure, heart attack, and stroke.

3. Restless leg syndrome: Restless leg syndrome is a neurological illness that produces an irrepressible impulse to move the legs, especially during the night. This can lead to problems falling asleep and daytime weariness.

4. Narcolepsy: Narcolepsy is like a mysterious thief who steals your wakefulness and leaves you powerless to resist its urges. It hits at any time,

without notice, making you feel like a puppet whose threads have been cut.Narcolepsy is an illness that involves extreme daytime sleepiness, sudden loss of muscle coordination, and sometimes hallucinations. This can greatly influence a person's capacity to operate during the day. Narcolepsy is like a mysterious thief that snatches your wakefulness and leaves you powerless to resist its whims. It hits at any time, without notice, making you feel like a puppet whose threads have been cut.

To manage various sleep disturbances, it is vital to first identify the underlying reason. In some circumstances, lifestyle changes such as maintaining a regular sleep schedule, avoiding caffeine and alcohol before bedtime, and practicing relaxation techniques like yoga or meditation can help improve sleep quality.

For more severe situations, medical treatment may be essential. For example, sleep apnea may be treated with a continuous positive airway pressure (CPAP) machine, while drugs may be used to treat insomnia or narcolepsy. A consultation with a sleep specialist or a healthcare professional can assist decide the most appropriate course of treatment.

Relaxation techniques for stress reduction and increased sleep

Stress is a prevalent issue that affects people of all ages and can lead to several health concerns such as anxiety, depression, and even cardiovascular illnesses. Additionally, stress can impair sleep, making it harder for individuals to get asleep, stay asleep, or obtain adequate restorative sleep. Relaxation techniques have been demonstrated to be useful in lowering stress levels and enhancing sleep quality. In this post, we will examine some of the most effective relaxation techniques for stress reduction and increased sleep.

1. Deep Breathing

Deep breathing is one of the easiest relaxing exercises to execute and can be done anywhere. It involves taking deep, slow breaths via the nose, holding the breath for a few seconds, then expelling slowly through the mouth. This approach helps to slow down the heart rate, relax the muscles, and quiet the mind.

To practice deep breathing, sit or lie down in a comfortable posture, close your eyes, and focus on your breath. Breathe deeply with your nose, filling your lungs with air, and then exhale slowly through your mouth. Repeat this procedure for a few minutes, focusing on the sensation of the breath traveling in and out of your body.

2. Progressive Muscle Relaxation

Progressive muscular relaxation is a technique that involves tensing and relaxing different muscle groups in the body to reduce muscle tension and promote relaxation. This approach is particularly effective for persons who keep a lot of tension in their muscles due to stress.

To practice progressive muscle relaxation, start by sitting or lying down in a comfortable position. Begin by tensing the muscles in your foot for a few seconds, then relax them. Move up to your calves, thighs, buttocks, belly, chest, arms, hands, neck, and face, tensing each muscle group for a few seconds before releasing the tension. Repeat the procedure for a few minutes, focusing on the sensation of relaxation in each muscle group.

3. Mindfulness Meditation

Mindfulness meditation is a practice that involves focusing on the present moment and accepting it without judgment. This approach can help reduce stress and enhance sleep quality by eliminating negative thoughts and encouraging relaxation.

To practice mindfulness meditation, choose a quiet location to sit or lie down in a comfortable position. Close your eyes and focus on your breath, directing your attention to the sensation of the breath traveling in and out of your body. If your mind wanders, softly bring your attention back to your breath without judgment. Repeat this method for a few minutes, gradually increasing the time of your meditation practice as you get more familiar with the technique.

4. Yoga

Yoga is a mind-body practice that incorporates a sequence of postures, breathing exercises, and meditation techniques. This method has been demonstrated to reduce stress levels and enhance sleep quality.

To practice yoga, select a class or online video that meets your skill and needs. Some pose that are particularly good for stress reduction and improved sleep include Child's Pose, Legs-Up-The-Wall Pose, and Corpse Pose.

5. Guided Imagery

Guided imagery is a relaxation technique that involves utilizing the imagination to create a serene and calming mental image. This technique can be beneficial in decreasing stress levels and fostering relaxation.

To practice guided imagery, locate a quiet spot to sit or lie down in a comfortable position. Close your eyes and visualize a serene and calming place, such as a beach or a forest. Visualize the details of this scenario, including the sounds, scents, and sensations. Stay with this image for a few minutes, allowing yourself to relax and let go of any stress or anxiety.

CHAPTER 6
BUILDING CONNECTIONS: RELATIONSHIPS AND COMMUNITY

The impact of positive relationships on overall health and wellbeing

Positive connections have a tremendous impact on overall health and wellness. Research has consistently demonstrated that persons who have positive interactions with others tend to be happier, healthier, and live longer than those who are socially isolated. In this post, we will study the impact of positive relationships on overall health and well-being, including physical health, mental health, and social health.

1. Physical Health: Positive relationships have been related to greater physical health outcomes. Studies have found that persons who have strong social networks and favorable relationships with others are less likely to suffer chronic health diseases such as

heart disease, stroke, and cancer. Additionally, excellent connections can contribute to a stronger immune system, improved sleep quality, and speedier recovery from illness or injury.

One reason for this is that positive connections might help reduce stress levels. When people feel socially supported, they are better able to manage stress and may experience fewer negative health effects as a result. Additionally, great connections can support healthy behaviors such as regular exercise, nutritious eating, and avoiding dangerous behaviors such as smoking or excessive drinking.

2. Mental Health: Positive connections can also have a big impact on mental health. People who have positive interactions with others tend to have better emotional well-being and are less likely to develop depression, anxiety, and other mental health illnesses.

One reason for this is that positive connections can create a sense of social support and connectedness. When people feel connected to others and have someone they can turn to for emotional support, they may be better able to manage stress and cope with challenging emotions. Additionally, positive connections can create a feeling of purpose and meaning in life, which can foster a sense of contentment and happiness.

3. Social Health: Positive interactions can also have a big impact on social health. People who have positive relationships with others tend to be more socially involved and have a higher sense of belonging within their society. This can lead to a better sense of identity and self-esteem.

Additionally, positive connections can create possibilities for personal growth and development. When people establish positive relationships with others, they may be exposed to new ideas, experiences, and viewpoints, which can widen their horizons and help them acquire new skills and interests.

Strategies for creating and maintaining healthy relationships

Building and maintaining healthy relationships takes time, effort, and attention. Whether it's a romantic partnership, friendship, or family relationship, the following tactics can assist ensure that the tie continues strong and fulfilling:

1. Communication: Effective communication is the cornerstone of any healthy relationship. It's crucial to be open, honest, and straightforward with your spouse, friend, or family member. Practice active listening and share your opinions and feelings clearly and politely. Also, be open to listening to their opinions and take their wants and feelings into account.

2. Trust: Trust is crucial in any relationship. Be consistent and reliable in your actions and words, and show that you can be counted on. Keep your promises and obligations, and be honest even when it's difficult. Trust is formed over time, and it can take just one act of dishonesty to lose it.

3. Respect: Treat your partner, friend, or family member with respect, especially through disputes or arguments. Respect their limits, ideas, and feelings, and avoid assaulting or ridiculing them. Remember that everyone has different opinions and experiences, and it's crucial to recognize and understand those differences.

4. Empathy: Empathy is the ability to comprehend and share the sentiments of others. It's crucial to put yourself in your spouse, friend, or family member's shoes and try to comprehend their perspective. This

can help you respond more compassionately and effectively to their wants and concerns.

5. Compromise: Relationships are about give-and-take. Be open to compromise and discover solutions that work for all parties. Focus on the wider picture and strive to establish common ground, even if you have different viewpoints or preferences.

6. Quality time: Spending quality time together is vital for creating and maintaining healthy relationships. Make time for each other, whether it's a date night, a phone call, or a family supper. Focus on being present and engaged during your time together, and try to minimize distractions.

7. Positivity: Positivity can assist build relationships and make them more enjoyable. Focus on the positive elements of your partner, friend, or family member, and praise their victories and

accomplishments. Show appreciation and gratitude for the little things they do, and strive to retain a cheerful mindset even during hard circumstances.

8. Forgiveness: Forgiveness is a crucial aspect of every healthy relationship. Everyone makes errors, and it's crucial to be able to forgive and move forward. Holding grudges or ruminating on past misdeeds can destroy relationships and inhibit growth and progress.

Finding support and community on your health journey

Finding support and community can have a dramatic impact on your health journey. Whether you are striving to adopt a better lifestyle, manage a chronic illness, or overcome a mental health difficulty, having a supportive network of individuals can make all the difference. Here are some ways in which establishing support and community can significantly impact your health journey:

1. Encouragement and Motivation: Being part of a supportive community can offer you encouragement and motivation to stick to your health goals. Knowing that you have people in your camp who believe in you and want to see you succeed can make it simpler to stay dedicated to your health journey.

2. Accountability: Having people who are holding you accountable can help keep you on track. When you are part of a group, you are more likely to follow through on your commitments and stay accountable to your health goals.

3. Shared Experiences: Being part of a community can provide you with the opportunity to share your experiences and learn from others. When you are coping with a health difficulty, it might be helpful to

know that you are not alone. Sharing your journey with others who understand what you are going through might make you feel less isolated and more connected.

4. Education and Information: Communities can be a fantastic source of education and information. You can learn from others who have been through similar health difficulties and get suggestions and advice on how to manage your health more efficiently. You can also remain up to date on the newest research and therapies in your profession.

5. Emotional Support: Health issues can be emotionally demanding, and having a supportive community can offer you the emotional support you need. When you are part of a community, you have individuals who are available to listen, offer advice, and provide a shoulder to lean on.

6. Improved Mental Health: Being part of a supportive community can have a good impact on your mental health. Studies have shown that social support can help lessen symptoms of anxiety and depression, boost self-esteem, and promote emotions of well-being and pleasure.

CHAPTER 7
CREATING A HEALTHY ENVIRONMENT: HOME AND WORKSPACES

Understanding the impact of your surroundings on your health

The environment we live in has a huge impact on our general health and well-being. Our environment encompasses the physical, social, and cultural settings in which we live, work, and play. From the air we breathe to the people we connect with; our surroundings can have both positive and bad effects on our health.

☐ Physical Environment:

The physical environment includes the natural and constructed surroundings in which we live. This can encompass our homes, companies, schools, parks, and communities. The physical environment can have a substantial impact on our health in the following ways:

a. Air quality: Poor air quality can have a significant impact on respiratory health, leading to asthma and other respiratory issues.

b. Water quality: Contaminated water can contribute to gastrointestinal disorders, such as diarrhea and other diseases.

c. Noise pollution: Exposure to loud noise can contribute to hearing loss and other health concerns, such as sleep disruptions, stress, and hypertension.

d. Green places: Access to green areas, such as parks, can boost mental health and physical activity levels.

e. Built environment: The design of buildings and localities can affect physical activity levels and access to healthy eating options.

☐ Social Environment:

The social environment encompasses the relationships we have with others and the social rules and values that impact our conduct. The social environment can have a substantial impact on our health in the following ways:

a. Social support: Strong social support networks can promote mental health, reduce stress, and improve overall health outcomes.

b. Social isolation: Lack of social support and social isolation can lead to poor mental health, depression, and other health problems.

c. Social norms: Social standards can influence health habits, such as smoking, alcohol consumption, and physical exercise.

d. prejudice: Experiencing prejudice can contribute to poor mental health and physical health effects.

☐ Cultural Environment:

The cultural environment includes the beliefs, values, and practices of our community and the greater society. The cultural environment can have a substantial impact on our health in the following ways:

a. Diet: Cultural ideas and practices can affect nutritional patterns, leading to either healthy or harmful food choices.

b. Health activities: Cultural norms can influence health behaviors, such as physical exercise and smoking.

c. Health literacy: Cultural differences in language, attitudes, and practices can impact health literacy, making it harder for individuals to receive and interpret health information.

d. Healthcare access: Cultural beliefs and practices can affect access to healthcare, leading to inequities in health outcomes.

In conclusion, our environment has a huge impact on our general health and well-being. Understanding the impact of our physical, social, and cultural surroundings can help us make educated decisions about our health and well-being. By building healthy environments that promote physical exercise, nutritious food choices, social support, and cultural knowledge, we can improve the health and well-being of individuals and communities.

Strategies for Creating a healthy home and Workspace

In today's fast-paced world, fostering a healthy and productive atmosphere is crucial for preserving physical and mental well-being. A healthy home and office not only enhances productivity but also reduces stress levels, boosts creativity, and encourages a good mindset. In this post, we will cover some of the ideas for having a healthy home and workspace.

The first and foremost tactic is to simplify and organize. Cluttered spaces can contribute to increased tension and anxiety, making it harder to focus on work or relax at home. Start with cleaning your home, getting rid of unneeded objects, and organizing your belongings. Invest in storage options such as shelves, baskets, and filing cabinets to keep your room tidy and clutter-free.

The second technique is to include natural components in your room. Natural light, plants, and fresh air can help reduce stress levels, boost mood, and promote productivity. Make sure to open windows periodically, allow natural light to come in, and add plants to your desk and house.

Another method is to create a designated workstation. Whether you work from home or have a home office, it's crucial to have a distinct workspace. This not only helps create a clear line between work and personal life but also increases focus and productivity. Choose a peaceful and well-lit environment, and invest in a comfortable desk and chair.

A healthy workstation and the house also require frequent cleaning and maintenance. Dust and grime can lead to allergies and respiratory difficulties, while an untidy area can inhibit productivity and increase stress levels. Develop a cleaning routine that suits your lifestyle, and make sure to keep your area tidy and well-maintained.

Another technique is to foster healthy habits. Incorporating healthy habits into your daily routine can help reduce stress levels and build a good mentality. Take regular breaks, perform deep breathing techniques, and prioritize self-care. This could involve frequent exercise, meditation, or other relaxing techniques.

Finally, it's necessary to create a helpful workplace. Surround yourself with good people who support your aims and aspirations. A friendly and supportive atmosphere can help reduce stress levels and foster a healthy mindset.

Conclusively, creating a healthy home and workstation demands a variety of measures. Decluttering, adding natural elements, having a designated workstation, regular cleaning and maintenance, promoting healthy habits, and creating a supportive environment are all vital for preserving physical and mental well-being. By applying these tactics, you may create a productive and positive workplace that fosters creativity, reduces stress levels, and supports a healthy lifestyle.

The relevance of sustainability and eco-conscious choices

Sustainability and eco-conscious decisions are becoming increasingly crucial in today's society, as we confront significant environmental concerns such as climate change and resource depletion. As individuals, we have a responsibility to make mindful decisions that encourage a healthy lifestyle, both for ourselves and for the planet. In this essay, we will examine the necessity of sustainability and eco-conscious choices for healthy living.

Firstly, sustainability and eco-conscious decisions encourage a healthier environment. By reducing our carbon footprint, conserving resources, and eliminating waste, we may help offset the negative impacts of climate change and reduce pollution. This not only benefits the globe but also enhances the quality of air, water, and soil that we rely on for our health and well-being. For example, opting to walk or bike instead of driving a car minimizes air pollution and encourages physical exercise, which can enhance cardiovascular health and reduce the risk of chronic diseases.

Secondly, sustainability and eco-conscious decisions might promote a better diet. By choosing foods that are sustainably grown and minimally processed, we may lessen our influence on the environment while simultaneously improving our health. For example, consuming a plant-based diet reduces greenhouse gas emissions and is associated with a lower risk of chronic diseases such as heart disease and cancer.

Thirdly, sustainability and eco-conscious decisions can foster a healthier home environment. By choosing non-toxic and ecologically friendly items, we can decrease our exposure to dangerous chemicals and contaminants. For example, adopting natural cleaning products and personal care goods might limit exposure to chemicals such as phthalates and parabens, which are connected with severe health impacts.

Fourthly, sustainability and eco-conscious choices can foster a healthy community. By supporting local companies and community projects that promote sustainability and environmental protection, we can contribute to a more resilient and thriving neighborhood. For example, supporting local farmers' markets not only provides access to fresh and healthy meals but also supports local farmers and minimizes the carbon footprint associated with the long-distance transportation of food.

Finally, sustainability and eco-conscious decisions can foster a healthier mindset. By making intentional decisions that correspond with our beliefs and support our well-being, we can build a sense of purpose and fulfillment. For example, participation in community activities or volunteering for environmental concerns can create a sense of connection and purpose, which is related to increased mental health and well-being.

CHAPTER 8
PUTTING IT ALL TOGETHER: CREATING YOUR PERSONALIZED HEALTH PLAN
Assessing your current health status and goals

Assessing your present health state is a vital first step toward achieving a healthy lifestyle. By taking the time to analyze where you are right now, you may find areas for growth and set realistic objectives for yourself.

To begin, consider scheduling a physical exam with your healthcare physician. This will provide you with a baseline assessment of your overall health, including any existing illnesses or risk factors. Your healthcare practitioner can also provide counseling on healthy habits and lifestyle adjustments that can help you attain your goals.

In addition to a physical assessment, you may wish to review your present routines and activities. Keep a notebook for a week or two and detail your food intake, exercise routine, and sleep patterns. This might help you identify places where you may need to make improvements.

Once you have a good grasp of your present health situation, you can begin to create goals for yourself. Be sure to make your goals explicit, quantifiable, and reachable. For example, rather than just declaring you want to "lose weight," define a goal of dropping a certain number of pounds within a certain timeframe.

It's also crucial to develop goals that correspond with your particular values and priorities. For example, if you value spending time with family and friends, establish a goal to combine physical activities that you can do together, such as hiking or playing a sport.

When it comes to reaching your goals, it's crucial to adopt a holistic approach. This includes focusing on several elements of your health, including nutrition, physical activity, sleep, stress management, and social interactions. It may be good to break down your goals into smaller, doable tasks and focus on making modest adjustments over time.

Finally, make sure to appreciate your victories along the road. Achieving a healthy lifestyle is a journey, and it's vital to recognize the progress you've made and the hard work you've put in. Whether it's treating yourself to a relaxing massage or celebrating with a healthy dinner, take the time to recognize and thank yourself for your work.

Factors to be considered while establishing a personal fitness program

When establishing a personal fitness program, numerous elements should be examined to ensure that the program is safe, effective, and suited to the individual's needs and goals. Here are some of the essential variables to consider:

a. Fitness goals: The first stage in establishing a fitness program is to determine the individual's goals, whether they are to lose weight, gain muscle, enhance endurance, or just maintain general health and fitness.

b. Fitness level: It's crucial to examine the individual's current fitness level and any limits or medical concerns they may have. This can help identify the proper amount of intensity and length for their workouts.

c. Time availability: The quantity of time available for exercise can also affect the design of a fitness program. It's crucial to establish a program that works into the individual's schedule and gives ample time to observe improvements.

d. Personal preferences: Consider the individual's preferences for types of exercise, such as strength training, cardio, or yoga. This can help keep kids motivated and involved in their workouts.

e. Nutrition: A well-rounded fitness program should also incorporate nutrition and food habits. This can help support the individual's fitness objectives and ensure they are feeding their body adequately for workouts.

f. Progress tracking: It's crucial to track progress regularly to see if the program is functioning and make adjustments as needed. This might assist keep the individual engaged and ensure they are making progress towards their goals.

By considering these characteristics, a personalized fitness program may be built that is safe, effective, and matched to the individual's needs and goals.

Setting achievable goals and action steps

Setting feasible goals and action stages is a critical aspect of creating a personalized health plan. By creating clear, quantifiable, and achievable goals, and breaking them down into small action stages, you can design a strategy that is personalized to your unique needs and lifestyle.

To begin, examine your present health status and your goal outcome. For example, if you are trying to reduce weight, your goal can be to shed 10 pounds during the following 3 months. Once you have a clear goal in mind, break it down into smaller, more doable action stages.

For example, your action actions might include: • Tracking your food intake for a week to discover areas where you can make healthier choices.

• Incorporating additional physical activity into your daily routine, such as taking a 30-minute walk each day.

• Drinking more water and limiting your intake of sugary beverages.

• Planning and preparing nutritious meals in advance to avoid harmful eating choices.

• Joining a support group or seeking the services of a personal trainer or nutritionist to stay motivated and on track.

It's crucial to note that everyone's health goals and action steps will be different based on their specific needs and lifestyle. Your personalized health plan should be suited to your circumstances and should be doable within a realistic timeframe.

In addition to creating clear goals and action actions, it's also crucial to track your progress and make adjustments as needed. Regularly analyzing your strategy and making changes when necessary can help you stay motivated and on track toward attaining your goals.

It's crucial to recognize the progress you've made and use your triumphs as an incentive to continue working towards your goals. By creating reasonable goals and breaking them down into small action stages, you can design a personalized health plan that works for you and helps you accomplish your intended outcomes.

Creating a long-term health plan for sustained success

Creating a long-term health strategy is vital for sustainable success. While short-term goals will help you make progress toward your intended outcomes, a long-term plan can help you build lasting habits and achieve sustainable results.

Here are some crucial steps to building a long-term health plan:

1. Define your vision: Start by identifying your long-term health goals. What do you want to achieve in terms of your health and well-being? What does success look like to you? Be explicit and make sure your goals connect with your values and priorities.

2. Break down your goals: Once you have a clear vision for your long-term health, break it down into

smaller, more doable goals. For example, if your long-term aim is to increase your general fitness, your short-term goals can include running a 5k race, lifting a certain amount of weight, or obtaining a specified level of flexibility.

3. Identify obstacles: Next, analyze what can stand in the way of attaining your goals. This can include physical constraints, lack of time or motivation, or other external impediments. By identifying potential hurdles beforehand, you may design a plan to overcome them and stay on course.

4. establish a plan: With your goals and challenges in mind, establish a clear plan for achieving sustained success. This could include adopting a daily or weekly routine that incorporates good behaviors like exercise, a healthy diet, and stress reduction. You can also consider receiving support from a coach, trainer, or healthcare expert to help you stay accountable and on track.

5. Track your progress: Regularly reviewing your progress can help you stay motivated and make modifications as needed. Use a notebook or monitoring tool to chronicle your exercises, meals, and other health-related activities. Celebrate your victories along the journey and embrace setbacks as chances to learn and improve.

6. Adjust your plan as needed: Over time, your health needs and goals may change. Be open to revising your plan as needed to ensure that it remains current and effective. Consult with a healthcare practitioner or other specialist if you need assistance or help.

Carrying out a long-term health strategy needs commitment, discipline, and patience. But by staying focused on your vision, breaking down your goals into achievable steps, and being adaptable in the face of hurdles and disappointments, you may achieve lasting success and create a healthier, happier life for yourself.

CONCLUSION

A healthy lifestyle is vital for general well-being and enjoyment. It's not simply about following a rigorous diet or exercise plan, but rather about building habits and making choices that support a healthy and full life.

Whether you are just starting on your journey to a healthy lifestyle, or you are seeking strategies to continue your progress and achieve long-term success, there are numerous tools and resources available to support you.

This book has provided a detailed guide to establishing a tailored health plan that fits your individual needs and lifestyle. By creating reasonable objectives, breaking them down into small action steps, and tracking your progress over time, you may achieve sustained success and create a healthier, happier life for yourself.

Remember, building a healthy lifestyle is not a one-time event, but rather an ongoing journey of learning, growth, and self-discovery. Be patient, stay committed, and appreciate your victories along the road. With the correct mindset, support, and tools, you can attain the healthy lifestyle you seek and deserve.